In Just 6 Weeks!

Better Body Journal for Women

Lose Weight & Feel Amazing
Turn Your "Before" Body Into "After"
Be More Confident
Have Success Without Stress

WENDY WALLACE

For more informat ion on this titles and our others, please visit us on the web at www.ScorpioMoon.com.

Scorpio Moon Publishing
Suite 264
2 Toronto St.
Toronto, ON Canada
M5C 2B5

Introduction

Welcome to the "In Just 6 Weeks" journal, and congratulations on taking the very first step towards a healthier and happier you!

Using this journal each day will help you achieve your weight loss goals and develop the kind of inner strength that comes from knowing that you have made the healthiest choices for you. You'll not only look better, but you'll also feel better, too!

We've all heard that weight loss comes down to the simple formula of "fewer calories in and more calories out." It seems really basic, and yet, so many of us who have tried to shed pounds know that the process of losing weight can be so much more involved.

Yes, eating less and moving more are vital to weight loss, but so is being aware of each positive change you make every step of the way. You've got to feel good about the progress you're making or your heart just won't be in it, and soon enough the old habits will creep back in and you'll be left wondering if you even have it in you to make the changes you so secretly desire. The truth is, you can—and with less effort than you might think.

Best of all, this journal wasn't created to give you more "work" to do or to burden you with another obligation that you feel you must fulfill. In fact, it will only take a few minutes each day.

I designed this journal to give you the opportunity to

keep track of the most important elements of your weight loss journey that will inspire the necessary confidence in you to keep going from day to day and week to week. Beyond ordinary trackers you may have used in the past, this journal will allow you to:

- Focus on all the things you did right each day
- Take better care of yourself than ever before
- Have a place to write how you feel about your progress
- Express gratitude for all the wonderful things in your life
- Stay on track with your daily, weekly, and master goals

After the six weeks has ended, you will have a book that you, yourself, have written. It will be a book detailing how you have come so far and changed your life for the better. It will be a book you can come back to time and time again to remind yourself of just how strong and committed you are and to be proud of the success you have achieved.

I wish you the best with all of the exciting and life-affirming changes you are about to make in your life.

Wendy Wallace
InJust6Weeks.com

How to Use This Journal

At the start of your six-week journey, be sure to weigh yourself and take your body measurements. Write them down on the *Beginning of This Journey* page. It is so important that you do this. It can be easy to get caught up in the daily ups and downs of staying on track while losing weight, and some days are better than others. By recording your actual weight and body measurements, you'll know just how far you've come and how much your devotion to staying on track has made a difference in the way you feel and how your body has changed by the time you come to the end of the journal.

TODAY, I ATE

While counting calories and documenting all that you eat can be beneficial to your weight loss effort, all that you need to do while using this journal is to ensure that you have at least one serving of each of the food group essentials that make up a healthy, well-balanced eating plan. With each meal, simply put a check mark in the circle to indicate you have made a positive choice:

lunch
   Ø 1-2 servings of fruit
      and/or veggies
   O 1 serving of whole grains
   Ø 1 serving of protein
   Ø drank water

To help you find a balance each day, try to tune into your own personal challenges. Be mindful of how often you ate, how you were able to stop eating once physically satisfied, how you stopped eating before bedtime, curtailed cravings at your desk during an afternoon slump, etc, Also, be sure to give yourself a daily, low-calorie treat. Knowing that you have not just eaten the right foods, but also took good care of yourself by fueling your body with regular meals, allowing it to rest, and enjoying one of your favorite foods in moderation is so vital to releasing weight from your body and keeping it off.

TODAY, I EXERCISED:

Consistency amid the hustle and bustle of daily life is the most important aspect of establishing better habits in our lives. The reality is, some days you won't have a lot of time to workout. However, finding even 15 minutes to move your body will not only make your body good, but you will also get the satisfaction of coming back to your journal and placing a check mark beside a time duration. You'll know that even during challenging days, you did your best. These challenging days will bridge you to the days when you are able to workout for 30–60 minutes (or more!) Your consistency with exercise will give you a sense of accomplishment and knowing you did something each day no matter what will fill you with personal pride.

today I exercised

O	✓	O	O	O
15 mins.	30 mins.	45 mins.	60 mins.	More!

Each day, take a minute to write about your workout. How you choose to detail your workout is completely up to you.

As an example you could write:

My workout was: *30 minutes on the treadmill and a yoga class*

Or...

My workout was: *Fantastic! For the first time in years, I was able to jog for 15 minutes without slowing down!*

MY WINS/MY STRUGGLES:

As you keep track of the time while you change your body, each day will come with successes and obstacles.

Each day, write your three "wins" for the day. Really take the time to think about all that you did right. Often times, we spend more time thinking about what we felt we didn't do right and why we didn't make better choices, and this can lead to abandoning the weight loss effort altogether. All the while, what we did do to take care of ourselves is easily forgotten. Remember your daily successes and celebrate them. It is the culmination of these successes—not your failures—that will lead to real weight loss.

my wins	my struggles
Went to the gym in the morning	*Didn't eat an afternoon snack*

That being said, it's essential to know which areas need improvement and be able to assess them objectively. Your "struggles" aren't meant to be reminders of what you "coulda/woulda/shoulda" done. Instead, write down the three behaviors that you feel need your attention. Don't beat yourself up over any obstacle or setback you face, and don't ignore it, either. Instead, write it down with the promise you will, gently and with a greater awareness, deal with it differently when the "struggle" comes up again. Lasting weight loss success is not about all-or-nothing behaviors. It takes time to modify behaviors and reactions to which you're accustomed.

TODAY, I TOOK CARE OF MYSELF BY:

Too often, we think of weight loss as being work that will eventually be rewarded, and we forget that the act of losing weight is really about taking good care of ourselves *now*. So many of us believe that we can only allow ourselves pleasurable things once we reach our goal weight, and so buying new clothes, finally going to a spa, or even just finally having the opportunity to be happy become mere fantasies that are pushed aside for a later date.

In your heart, you know you are doing yourself a disservice by putting off self-care until the future. You need to be doing things, even small, simple things, to take care of and replenish yourself right now. Each day commit to doing four things to take care of yourself. Each act of self-love can be something as effortless as taking a nap or sitting quietly for a while, or getting out and doing enjoyable things like shopping at a bookstore or meeting up with a friend.

*Took a break from work
& went to a movie*

HOW I AM FEELING TODAY:

In this section of your journal, you are free to express your-self whichever way you choose. You may want to write out the emotions you are feeling in full sentences or sum things up in one word, written in large capital letters. Or, perhaps you'll want to express yourself with a drawing or doodles. Take the space to just let loose and put your feelings on paper.

how I am feeling today . . .

It was an incredible day! I'm really tired, but I feel good about the workout I did today.

TODAY, I AM GRATEFUL FOR:

Losing weight can sometimes feel like an uphill struggle, but if you always keep in mind the wonderful things already in your life each day, and look forward to new, unexpected surprises, you will make your life that much better. Take time everyday to write five things that you are grateful for. Doing so will bring you back to feelings of love and appre-ciation for your life and yourself. While eating right and exercising are crucial, developing a state of gratitude can help make your weight loss journey unfold tremendously easier and faster.

today, I am grateful for

Having access to fresh, healthy food

DAILY INTENTIONS:

Finally, as you wrap up each day, spend some time thinking about tomorrow.

In the midst of losing weight, sometimes, we lose sight of why we are doing it. Have you ever been in a restaurant and found yourself wanting to order french fries or a decadent dessert, despite being full from your meal? In your mind, a battle begins between wanting to experience the enjoyment you remember getting out of eating fries or sweets and knowing that doing so will take you a small step back from your weight loss goal. During times like these, your desire to accomplish your goal has to be stronger than the desire to indulge.

The way to keep your desire to lose weight strong and at the forefront of your mind to battle in-the-moment cravings is to write out your intentions each day.

In this section, you will write your intention for the following day and describe how it will help you achieve your weekly and master goals.

For example:

My intention for tomorrow is: to go for a 30-minute walk

...which helps me reach my weekly goal of: losing 2 pounds

...which helps me reach my master goal of: being able to fit into the jeans I haven't worn in five years

> *my intention for tomorrow is:*
>
> Add five more minutes to my cardio workout

At the end of the six weeks, once again, on the *How Far I've Come!* page, write down your current weight and your measurements. Now, step back and look at how far you have come! Being able to see that all of your efforts to be good to yourself paid off will not only offer a huge boost to your self-confidence, but it will be enough to take you into the next six weeks, if you have more weight to lose.

And if you have more to lose, don't fret. Even if your weight loss goals continue beyond six weeks, knowing you have completed this journal is a testament of how much you care about yourself, how much you want a better life, and that you are capable of having all that you want.

If you would like to receive daily motivation, support from others who are using the "In Just 6 Weeks" journal, and receive free journal updates, please visit: InJust6Weeks.com

The Beginning of This Journey

my current weight _____

my current measurements:

Left arm: _____

Right arm: _____

Chest: _____

Waist: _____

Hips: _____

Left thigh: _____

Right thigh: _____

in six weeks, I see myself being:

Week 1, Day 1

today I ate

breakfast
- ○ 1-2 servings of fruit and/or veggies
- ○ 1 serving of whole grains
- ○ 1 serving of protein
- ○ drank water

snack
- ○ 1-2 servings of fruit and/or veggies
- ○ 1 serving of whole grains
- ○ 1 serving of protein
- ○ drank water

lunch
- ○ 1-2 servings of fruit and/or veggies
- ○ 1 serving of whole grains
- ○ 1 serving of protein
- ○ drank water

snack
- ○ 1-2 servings of fruit and/or veggies
- ○ 1 serving of whole grains
- ○ 1 serving of protein
- ○ drank water

dinner
- ○ 1-2 servings of fruit and/or veggies
- ○ 1 serving of whole grains
- ○ 1 serving of protein
- ○ drank water

snack
- ○ 1-2 servings of fruit and/or veggies
- ○ 1 serving of whole grains
- ○ 1 serving of protein
- ○ drank water

- ○ Ate every 2-3 hours
- ○ Stopped eating 3 hours before bed
- ○ Allowed myself 1 small treat (300 calories or less)

today I exercised

○ 15 mins.   ○ 30 mins.   ○ 45 mins.   ○ 60 mins.   ○ More!

my workout was: _____

_____

Week 1, Day 1

my wins

_____

_____

_____

my struggles

_____

_____

_____

I took care of myself by

Week 1, Day 1

how I am feeling today . . .

today, I am grateful for

_____

_____

_____

_____

_____

my intention for tomorrow is:

. . . which helps me reach my weekly goal of:

. . . and helps me reach my master goal of:

my intention for tomorrow is:

. . . which helps me reach my weekly goal of:

. . . and helps me reach my master goal of:

my intention for tomorrow is:

. . . which helps me reach my weekly goal of:

. . . and helps me reach my master goal of:

Week 1, Day 2

today I ate

breakfast
- ○ 1-2 servings of fruit and/or veggies
- ○ 1 serving of whole grains
- ○ 1 serving of protein
- ○ drank water

snack
- ○ 1-2 servings of fruit and/or veggies
- ○ 1 serving of whole grains
- ○ 1 serving of protein
- ○ drank water

lunch
- ○ 1-2 servings of fruit and/or veggies
- ○ 1 serving of whole grains
- ○ 1 serving of protein
- ○ drank water

snack
- ○ 1-2 servings of fruit and/or veggies
- ○ 1 serving of whole grains
- ○ 1 serving of protein
- ○ drank water

dinner
- ○ 1-2 servings of fruit and/or veggies
- ○ 1 serving of whole grains
- ○ 1 serving of protein
- ○ drank water

snack
- ○ 1-2 servings of fruit and/or veggies
- ○ 1 serving of whole grains
- ○ 1 serving of protein
- ○ drank water

- ○ Ate every 2-3 hours
- ○ Stopped eating 3 hours before bed
- ○ Allowed myself 1 small treat (300 calories or less)

today I exercised

○ 15 mins.   ○ 30 mins.   ○ 45 mins.   ○ 60 mins.   ○ More!

my workout was: _____

_____

my wins

_____

_____

_____

my struggles

_____

_____

_____

I took care of myself by

how I am feeling today . . .

today, I am grateful for

_____

_____

_____

_____

_____

my intention for tomorrow is:

. . . which helps me reach my weekly goal of:

. . . and helps me reach my master goal of:

my intention for tomorrow is:

. . . which helps me reach my weekly goal of:

. . . and helps me reach my master goal of:

my intention for tomorrow is:

. . . which helps me reach my weekly goal of:

. . . and helps me reach my master goal of:

today I ate

breakfast
- ○ 1-2 servings of fruit and/or veggies
- ○ 1 serving of whole grains
- ○ 1 serving of protein
- ○ drank water

snack
- ○ 1-2 servings of fruit and/or veggies
- ○ 1 serving of whole grains
- ○ 1 serving of protein
- ○ drank water

lunch
- ○ 1-2 servings of fruit and/or veggies
- ○ 1 serving of whole grains
- ○ 1 serving of protein
- ○ drank water

snack
- ○ 1-2 servings of fruit and/or veggies
- ○ 1 serving of whole grains
- ○ 1 serving of protein
- ○ drank water

dinner
- ○ 1-2 servings of fruit and/or veggies
- ○ 1 serving of whole grains
- ○ 1 serving of protein
- ○ drank water

snack
- ○ 1-2 servings of fruit and/or veggies
- ○ 1 serving of whole grains
- ○ 1 serving of protein
- ○ drank water

- ○ Ate every 2-3 hours
- ○ Stopped eating 3 hours before bed
- ○ Allowed myself 1 small treat (300 calories or less)

today I exercised

○ 15 mins. ○ 30 mins. ○ 45 mins. ○ 60 mins. ○ More!

my workout was: _____

_____

Week 1, Day 3

my wins

_____

_____

_____

my struggles

_____

_____

_____

I took care of myself by

how I am feeling today . . .

today, I am grateful for

_____

_____

_____

_____

_____

my intention for tomorrow is:

. . . which helps me reach my weekly goal of:

. . . and helps me reach my master goal of:

my intention for tomorrow is:

. . . which helps me reach my weekly goal of:

. . . and helps me reach my master goal of:

my intention for tomorrow is:

. . . which helps me reach my weekly goal of:

. . . and helps me reach my master goal of:

Week 1, Day 4

today I ate

breakfast
- ○ 1-2 servings of fruit and/or veggies
- ○ 1 serving of whole grains
- ○ 1 serving of protein
- ○ drank water

snack
- ○ 1-2 servings of fruit and/or veggies
- ○ 1 serving of whole grains
- ○ 1 serving of protein
- ○ drank water

snack
- ○ 1-2 servings of fruit and/or veggies
- ○ 1 serving of whole grains
- ○ 1 serving of protein
- ○ drank water

dinner
- ○ 1-2 servings of fruit and/or veggies
- ○ 1 serving of whole grains
- ○ 1 serving of protein
- ○ drank water

lunch
- ○ 1-2 servings of fruit and/or veggies
- ○ 1 serving of whole grains
- ○ 1 serving of protein
- ○ drank water

snack
- ○ 1-2 servings of fruit and/or veggies
- ○ 1 serving of whole grains
- ○ 1 serving of protein
- ○ drank water

- ○ Ate every 2-3 hours
- ○ Stopped eating 3 hours before bed
- ○ Allowed myself 1 small treat (300 calories or less)

today I exercised

○ 15 mins.　　○ 30 mins.　　○ 45 mins.　　○ 60 mins.　　○ More!

my workout was: _____

_____

Week 1, Day 4

my wins

_____

_____

_____

my struggles

_____

_____

_____

I took care of myself by

how I am feeling today . . .

today, I am grateful for

_____

_____

_____

_____

_____

my intention for tomorrow is:

. . . which helps me reach my weekly goal of:

. . . and helps me reach my master goal of:

my intention for tomorrow is:

. . . which helps me reach my weekly goal of:

. . . and helps me reach my master goal of:

my intention for tomorrow is:

. . . which helps me reach my weekly goal of:

. . . and helps me reach my master goal of:

Week 1, Day 5

today I ate

breakfast
- O 1-2 servings of fruit and/or veggies
- O 1 serving of whole grains
- O 1 serving of protein
- O drank water

snack
- O 1-2 servings of fruit and/or veggies
- O 1 serving of whole grains
- O 1 serving of protein
- O drank water

lunch
- O 1-2 servings of fruit and/or veggies
- O 1 serving of whole grains
- O 1 serving of protein
- O drank water

snack
- O 1-2 servings of fruit and/or veggies
- O 1 serving of whole grains
- O 1 serving of protein
- O drank water

dinner
- O 1-2 servings of fruit and/or veggies
- O 1 serving of whole grains
- O 1 serving of protein
- O drank water

snack
- O 1-2 servings of fruit and/or veggies
- O 1 serving of whole grains
- O 1 serving of protein
- O drank water

O Ate every 2-3 hours
O Stopped eating 3 hours before bed
O Allowed myself 1 small treat (300 calories or less)

today I exercised

O 15 mins.   O 30 mins.   O 45 mins.   O 60 mins.   O More!

my workout was: _____

_____

Week 1, Day 5

my wins

_____

_____

_____

my struggles

_____

_____

_____

I took care of myself by

Week 1, Day 5

how I am feeling today . . .

today, I am grateful for

_____

_____

_____

_____

_____

my intention for tomorrow is:

. . . which helps me reach my weekly goal of:

. . . and helps me reach my master goal of:

my intention for tomorrow is:

. . . which helps me reach my weekly goal of:

. . . and helps me reach my master goal of:

my intention for tomorrow is:

. . . which helps me reach my weekly goal of:

. . . and helps me reach my master goal of:

Week 1, Day 6

today I ate

breakfast
- ○ 1-2 servings of fruit and/or veggies
- ○ 1 serving of whole grains
- ○ 1 serving of protein
- ○ drank water

snack
- ○ 1-2 servings of fruit and/or veggies
- ○ 1 serving of whole grains
- ○ 1 serving of protein
- ○ drank water

lunch
- ○ 1-2 servings of fruit and/or veggies
- ○ 1 serving of whole grains
- ○ 1 serving of protein
- ○ drank water

snack
- ○ 1-2 servings of fruit and/or veggies
- ○ 1 serving of whole grains
- ○ 1 serving of protein
- ○ drank water

dinner
- ○ 1-2 servings of fruit and/or veggies
- ○ 1 serving of whole grains
- ○ 1 serving of protein
- ○ drank water

snack
- ○ 1-2 servings of fruit and/or veggies
- ○ 1 serving of whole grains
- ○ 1 serving of protein
- ○ drank water

- ○ Ate every 2-3 hours
- ○ Stopped eating 3 hours before bed
- ○ Allowed myself 1 small treat (300 calories or less)

today I exercised

○ 15 mins. ○ 30 mins. ○ 45 mins. ○ 60 mins. ○ More!

my workout was: _____

_____

my wins

_____

_____

_____

my struggles

_____

_____

_____

I took care of myself by

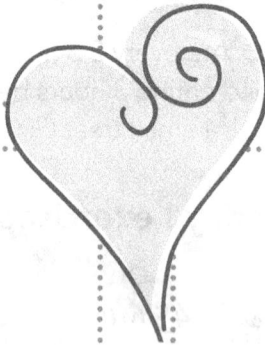

how I am feeling today . . .

today, I am grateful for

_____

_____

_____

_____

_____

my intention for tomorrow is:

. . . which helps me reach my weekly goal of:

. . . and helps me reach my master goal of:

my intention for tomorrow is:

. . . which helps me reach my weekly goal of:

. . . and helps me reach my master goal of:

my intention for tomorrow is:

. . . which helps me reach my weekly goal of:

. . . and helps me reach my master goal of:

Week 1, Day 7

today I ate

breakfast
- ○ 1-2 servings of fruit and/or veggies
- ○ 1 serving of whole grains
- ○ 1 serving of protein
- ○ drank water

snack
- ○ 1-2 servings of fruit and/or veggies
- ○ 1 serving of whole grains
- ○ 1 serving of protein
- ○ drank water

lunch
- ○ 1-2 servings of fruit and/or veggies
- ○ 1 serving of whole grains
- ○ 1 serving of protein
- ○ drank water

snack
- ○ 1-2 servings of fruit and/or veggies
- ○ 1 serving of whole grains
- ○ 1 serving of protein
- ○ drank water

dinner
- ○ 1-2 servings of fruit and/or veggies
- ○ 1 serving of whole grains
- ○ 1 serving of protein
- ○ drank water

snack
- ○ 1-2 servings of fruit and/or veggies
- ○ 1 serving of whole grains
- ○ 1 serving of protein
- ○ drank water

- ○ Ate every 2-3 hours
- ○ Stopped eating 3 hours before bed
- ○ Allowed myself 1 small treat (300 calories or less)

today I exercised

○ 15 mins.   ○ 30 mins.   ○ 45 mins.   ○ 60 mins.   ○ More!

my workout was: _____

_____

my wins

my struggles

_____

_____

_____

_____

_____

_____

I took care of myself by

Week 1, Day 7

how I am feeling today . . .

today, I am grateful for

_____

_____

_____

_____

_____

my intention for tomorrow is:

. . . which helps me reach my weekly goal of:

. . . and helps me reach my master goal of:

my intention for tomorrow is:

. . . which helps me reach my weekly goal of:

. . . and helps me reach my master goal of:

my intention for tomorrow is:

. . . which helps me reach my weekly goal of:

. . . and helps me reach my master goal of:

Week 2, Day 1

today I ate

breakfast
- ○ 1-2 servings of fruit and/or veggies
- ○ 1 serving of whole grains
- ○ 1 serving of protein
- ○ drank water

snack
- ○ 1-2 servings of fruit and/or veggies
- ○ 1 serving of whole grains
- ○ 1 serving of protein
- ○ drank water

lunch
- ○ 1-2 servings of fruit and/or veggies
- ○ 1 serving of whole grains
- ○ 1 serving of protein
- ○ drank water

snack
- ○ 1-2 servings of fruit and/or veggies
- ○ 1 serving of whole grains
- ○ 1 serving of protein
- ○ drank water

dinner
- ○ 1-2 servings of fruit and/or veggies
- ○ 1 serving of whole grains
- ○ 1 serving of protein
- ○ drank water

snack
- ○ 1-2 servings of fruit and/or veggies
- ○ 1 serving of whole grains
- ○ 1 serving of protein
- ○ drank water

- ○ Ate every 2-3 hours
- ○ Stopped eating 3 hours before bed
- ○ Allowed myself 1 small treat (300 calories or less)

today I exercised

○ 15 mins. ○ 30 mins. ○ 45 mins. ○ 60 mins. ○ More!

my workout was: _____

_____

Week 2, Day 1

my wins

_____

_____

_____

my struggles

_____

_____

_____

I took care of myself by

how I am feeling today . . .

today, I am grateful for

_____

_____

_____

_____

_____

my intention for tomorrow is:

. . . which helps me reach my weekly goal of:

. . . and helps me reach my master goal of:

my intention for tomorrow is:

. . . which helps me reach my weekly goal of:

. . . and helps me reach my master goal of:

my intention for tomorrow is:

. . . which helps me reach my weekly goal of:

. . . and helps me reach my master goal of:

Week 2, Day 2

today I ate

breakfast
- ○ 1-2 servings of fruit and/or veggies
- ○ 1 serving of whole grains
- ○ 1 serving of protein
- ○ drank water

snack
- ○ 1-2 servings of fruit and/or veggies
- ○ 1 serving of whole grains
- ○ 1 serving of protein
- ○ drank water

lunch
- ○ 1-2 servings of fruit and/or veggies
- ○ 1 serving of whole grains
- ○ 1 serving of protein
- ○ drank water

snack
- ○ 1-2 servings of fruit and/or veggies
- ○ 1 serving of whole grains
- ○ 1 serving of protein
- ○ drank water

dinner
- ○ 1-2 servings of fruit and/or veggies
- ○ 1 serving of whole grains
- ○ 1 serving of protein
- ○ drank water

snack
- ○ 1-2 servings of fruit and/or veggies
- ○ 1 serving of whole grains
- ○ 1 serving of protein
- ○ drank water

- ○ Ate every 2-3 hours
- ○ Stopped eating 3 hours before bed
- ○ Allowed myself 1 small treat (300 calories or less)

today I exercised

○ 15 mins.   ○ 30 mins.   ○ 45 mins.   ○ 60 mins.   ○ More!

my workout was: _____

_____

Week 2, Day 2

my wins

_____

_____

_____

🌿

my struggles

_____

_____

_____

🌿

I took care of myself by

48

how I am feeling today . . .

today, I am grateful for

_____

_____

_____

_____

_____

my intention for tomorrow is:

. . . which helps me reach my weekly goal of:

. . . and helps me reach my master goal of:

my intention for tomorrow is:

. . . which helps me reach my weekly goal of:

. . . and helps me reach my master goal of:

my intention for tomorrow is:

. . . which helps me reach my weekly goal of:

. . . and helps me reach my master goal of:

Week 2, Day 3

today I ate

breakfast
- ○ 1-2 servings of fruit and/or veggies
- ○ 1 serving of whole grains
- ○ 1 serving of protein
- ○ drank water

snack
- ○ 1-2 servings of fruit and/or veggies
- ○ 1 serving of whole grains
- ○ 1 serving of protein
- ○ drank water

lunch
- ○ 1-2 servings of fruit and/or veggies
- ○ 1 serving of whole grains
- ○ 1 serving of protein
- ○ drank water

snack
- ○ 1-2 servings of fruit and/or veggies
- ○ 1 serving of whole grains
- ○ 1 serving of protein
- ○ drank water

dinner
- ○ 1-2 servings of fruit and/or veggies
- ○ 1 serving of whole grains
- ○ 1 serving of protein
- ○ drank water

snack
- ○ 1-2 servings of fruit and/or veggies
- ○ 1 serving of whole grains
- ○ 1 serving of protein
- ○ drank water

- ○ Ate every 2-3 hours
- ○ Stopped eating 3 hours before bed
- ○ Allowed myself 1 small treat (300 calories or less)

today I exercised

○ 15 mins.   ○ 30 mins.   ○ 45 mins.   ○ 60 mins.   ○ More!

my workout was: _____

_____

Week 2, Day 3

my wins

_____

_____

_____

my struggles

_____

_____

_____

I took care of myself by

Week 2, Day 3

how I am feeling today . . .

today, I am grateful for

_____

_____

_____

_____

_____

my intention for tomorrow is:

. . . which helps me reach my weekly goal of:

. . . and helps me reach my master goal of:

my intention for tomorrow is:

. . . which helps me reach my weekly goal of:

. . . and helps me reach my master goal of:

my intention for tomorrow is:

. . . which helps me reach my weekly goal of:

. . . and helps me reach my master goal of:

Week 2, Day 4

breakfast
- ○ 1-2 servings of fruit and/or veggies
- ○ 1 serving of whole grains
- ○ 1 serving of protein
- ○ drank water

snack
- ○ 1-2 servings of fruit and/or veggies
- ○ 1 serving of whole grains
- ○ 1 serving of protein
- ○ drank water

lunch
- ○ 1-2 servings of fruit and/or veggies
- ○ 1 serving of whole grains
- ○ 1 serving of protein
- ○ drank water

today I ate

snack
- ○ 1-2 servings of fruit and/or veggies
- ○ 1 serving of whole grains
- ○ 1 serving of protein
- ○ drank water

dinner
- ○ 1-2 servings of fruit and/or veggies
- ○ 1 serving of whole grains
- ○ 1 serving of protein
- ○ drank water

snack
- ○ 1-2 servings of fruit and/or veggies
- ○ 1 serving of whole grains
- ○ 1 serving of protein
- ○ drank water

- ○ Ate every 2-3 hours
- ○ Stopped eating 3 hours before bed
- ○ Allowed myself 1 small treat (300 calories or less)

today I exercised

○	○	○	○	○
15 mins.	30 mins.	45 mins.	60 mins.	More!

my workout was: _____

_____

my wins

_____

_____

_____

my struggles

_____

_____

_____

I took care of myself by

how I am feeling today . . .

today, I am grateful for

_____

_____

_____

_____

_____

my intention for tomorrow is:

. . . which helps me reach my weekly goal of:

. . . and helps me reach my master goal of:

my intention for tomorrow is:

. . . which helps me reach my weekly goal of:

. . . and helps me reach my master goal of:

my intention for tomorrow is:

. . . which helps me reach my weekly goal of:

. . . and helps me reach my master goal of:

Week 2, Day 5

today I ate

breakfast
- ○ 1-2 servings of fruit and/or veggies
- ○ 1 serving of whole grains
- ○ 1 serving of protein
- ○ drank water

snack
- ○ 1-2 servings of fruit and/or veggies
- ○ 1 serving of whole grains
- ○ 1 serving of protein
- ○ drank water

lunch
- ○ 1-2 servings of fruit and/or veggies
- ○ 1 serving of whole grains
- ○ 1 serving of protein
- ○ drank water

snack
- ○ 1-2 servings of fruit and/or veggies
- ○ 1 serving of whole grains
- ○ 1 serving of protein
- ○ drank water

dinner
- ○ 1-2 servings of fruit and/or veggies
- ○ 1 serving of whole grains
- ○ 1 serving of protein
- ○ drank water

snack
- ○ 1-2 servings of fruit and/or veggies
- ○ 1 serving of whole grains
- ○ 1 serving of protein
- ○ drank water

- ○ Ate every 2-3 hours
- ○ Stopped eating 3 hours before bed
- ○ Allowed myself 1 small treat (300 calories or less)

today I exercised

○ 15 mins.   ○ 30 mins.   ○ 45 mins.   ○ 60 mins.   ○ More!

my workout was: _____

_____

Week 2, Day 5

my wins

_____
_____
_____

my struggles

_____
_____
_____

I took care of myself by

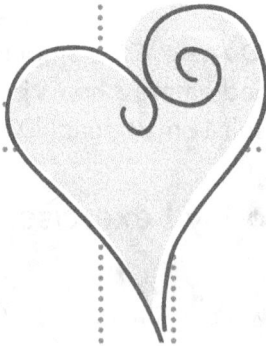

Week 2, Day 5

how I am feeling today . . .

today, I am grateful for

_____

_____

_____

_____

_____

my intention for tomorrow is:

. . . which helps me reach my weekly goal of:

. . . and helps me reach my master goal of:

my intention for tomorrow is:

. . . which helps me reach my weekly goal of:

. . . and helps me reach my master goal of:

my intention for tomorrow is:

. . . which helps me reach my weekly goal of:

. . . and helps me reach my master goal of:

Week 2, Day 6

today I ate

breakfast
- ○ 1-2 servings of fruit and/or veggies
- ○ 1 serving of whole grains
- ○ 1 serving of protein
- ○ drank water

snack
- ○ 1-2 servings of fruit and/or veggies
- ○ 1 serving of whole grains
- ○ 1 serving of protein
- ○ drank water

lunch
- ○ 1-2 servings of fruit and/or veggies
- ○ 1 serving of whole grains
- ○ 1 serving of protein
- ○ drank water

snack
- ○ 1-2 servings of fruit and/or veggies
- ○ 1 serving of whole grains
- ○ 1 serving of protein
- ○ drank water

dinner
- ○ 1-2 servings of fruit and/or veggies
- ○ 1 serving of whole grains
- ○ 1 serving of protein
- ○ drank water

snack
- ○ 1-2 servings of fruit and/or veggies
- ○ 1 serving of whole grains
- ○ 1 serving of protein
- ○ drank water

- ○ Ate every 2-3 hours
- ○ Stopped eating 3 hours before bed
- ○ Allowed myself 1 small treat (300 calories or less)

today I exercised

○ 15 mins.   ○ 30 mins.   ○ 45 mins.   ○ 60 mins.   ○ More!

my workout was: _____

_____

Week 2, Day 6

my wins

my struggles

I took care of myself by

how I am feeling today . . .

today, I am grateful for

_____

_____

_____

_____

_____

my intention for tomorrow is:

. . . which helps me reach my weekly goal of:

. . . and helps me reach my master goal of:

my intention for tomorrow is:

. . . which helps me reach my weekly goal of:

. . . and helps me reach my master goal of:

my intention for tomorrow is:

. . . which helps me reach my weekly goal of:

. . . and helps me reach my master goal of:

Week 2, Day 7

today I ate

breakfast
- ○ 1-2 servings of fruit and/or veggies
- ○ 1 serving of whole grains
- ○ 1 serving of protein
- ○ drank water

snack
- ○ 1-2 servings of fruit and/or veggies
- ○ 1 serving of whole grains
- ○ 1 serving of protein
- ○ drank water

lunch
- ○ 1-2 servings of fruit and/or veggies
- ○ 1 serving of whole grains
- ○ 1 serving of protein
- ○ drank water

snack
- ○ 1-2 servings of fruit and/or veggies
- ○ 1 serving of whole grains
- ○ 1 serving of protein
- ○ drank water

dinner
- ○ 1-2 servings of fruit and/or veggies
- ○ 1 serving of whole grains
- ○ 1 serving of protein
- ○ drank water

snack
- ○ 1-2 servings of fruit and/or veggies
- ○ 1 serving of whole grains
- ○ 1 serving of protein
- ○ drank water

- ○ Ate every 2-3 hours
- ○ Stopped eating 3 hours before bed
- ○ Allowed myself 1 small treat (300 calories or less)

today I exercised

○ 15 mins.   ○ 30 mins.   ○ 45 mins.   ○ 60 mins.   ○ More!

my workout was: _____

my wins

_____

_____

_____

my struggles

_____

_____

_____

I took care of myself by

Week 2, Day 7

how I am feeling today . . .

today, I am grateful for

_____

_____

_____

_____

_____

my intention for tomorrow is:

. . . which helps me reach my weekly goal of:

. . . and helps me reach my master goal of:

my intention for tomorrow is:

. . . which helps me reach my weekly goal of:

. . . and helps me reach my master goal of:

my intention for tomorrow is:

. . . which helps me reach my weekly goal of:

. . . and helps me reach my master goal of:

Week 3, Day 1

today I ate

breakfast
- ○ 1-2 servings of fruit and/or veggies
- ○ 1 serving of whole grains
- ○ 1 serving of protein
- ○ drank water

snack
- ○ 1-2 servings of fruit and/or veggies
- ○ 1 serving of whole grains
- ○ 1 serving of protein
- ○ drank water

lunch
- ○ 1-2 servings of fruit and/or veggies
- ○ 1 serving of whole grains
- ○ 1 serving of protein
- ○ drank water

snack
- ○ 1-2 servings of fruit and/or veggies
- ○ 1 serving of whole grains
- ○ 1 serving of protein
- ○ drank water

dinner
- ○ 1-2 servings of fruit and/or veggies
- ○ 1 serving of whole grains
- ○ 1 serving of protein
- ○ drank water

snack
- ○ 1-2 servings of fruit and/or veggies
- ○ 1 serving of whole grains
- ○ 1 serving of protein
- ○ drank water

- ○ Ate every 2-3 hours
- ○ Stopped eating 3 hours before bed
- ○ Allowed myself 1 small treat (300 calories or less)

today I exercised

○	○	○	○	○
15 mins.	30 mins.	45 mins.	60 mins.	More!

my workout was: _____

_____

Week 3, Day 1

my wins

_____

_____

_____

my struggles

_____

_____

_____

I took care of myself by

Week 3, Day 1

how I am feeling today . . .

today, I am grateful for

_____

_____

_____

_____

_____

73

my intention for tomorrow is:

. . . which helps me reach my weekly goal of:

. . . and helps me reach my master goal of:

my intention for tomorrow is:

. . . which helps me reach my weekly goal of:

. . . and helps me reach my master goal of:

my intention for tomorrow is:

. . . which helps me reach my weekly goal of:

. . . and helps me reach my master goal of:

today I ate

breakfast
- ○ 1-2 servings of fruit and/or veggies
- ○ 1 serving of whole grains
- ○ 1 serving of protein
- ○ drank water

snack
- ○ 1-2 servings of fruit and/or veggies
- ○ 1 serving of whole grains
- ○ 1 serving of protein
- ○ drank water

lunch
- ○ 1-2 servings of fruit and/or veggies
- ○ 1 serving of whole grains
- ○ 1 serving of protein
- ○ drank water

snack
- ○ 1-2 servings of fruit and/or veggies
- ○ 1 serving of whole grains
- ○ 1 serving of protein
- ○ drank water

dinner
- ○ 1-2 servings of fruit and/or veggies
- ○ 1 serving of whole grains
- ○ 1 serving of protein
- ○ drank water

snack
- ○ 1-2 servings of fruit and/or veggies
- ○ 1 serving of whole grains
- ○ 1 serving of protein
- ○ drank water

- ○ Ate every 2-3 hours
- ○ Stopped eating 3 hours before bed
- ○ Allowed myself 1 small treat (300 calories or less)

today I exercised

○ 15 mins.   ○ 30 mins.   ○ 45 mins.   ○ 60 mins.   ○ More!

my workout was: _____

_____

my wins

_____

_____

_____

my struggles

_____

_____

_____

I took care of myself by

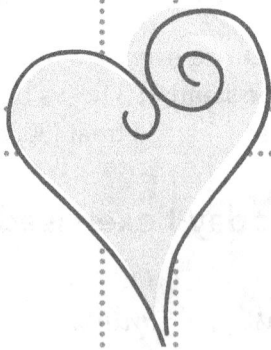

how I am feeling today . . .

today, I am grateful for

_____

_____

_____

_____

_____

my intention for tomorrow is:

. . . which helps me reach my weekly goal of:

. . . and helps me reach my master goal of:

my intention for tomorrow is:

. . . which helps me reach my weekly goal of:

. . . and helps me reach my master goal of:

my intention for tomorrow is:

. . . which helps me reach my weekly goal of:

. . . and helps me reach my master goal of:

today I ate

breakfast
- ○ 1-2 servings of fruit and/or veggies
- ○ 1 serving of whole grains
- ○ 1 serving of protein
- ○ drank water

snack
- ○ 1-2 servings of fruit and/or veggies
- ○ 1 serving of whole grains
- ○ 1 serving of protein
- ○ drank water

lunch
- ○ 1-2 servings of fruit and/or veggies
- ○ 1 serving of whole grains
- ○ 1 serving of protein
- ○ drank water

snack
- ○ 1-2 servings of fruit and/or veggies
- ○ 1 serving of whole grains
- ○ 1 serving of protein
- ○ drank water

dinner
- ○ 1-2 servings of fruit and/or veggies
- ○ 1 serving of whole grains
- ○ 1 serving of protein
- ○ drank water

snack
- ○ 1-2 servings of fruit and/or veggies
- ○ 1 serving of whole grains
- ○ 1 serving of protein
- ○ drank water

- ○ Ate every 2-3 hours
- ○ Stopped eating 3 hours before bed
- ○ Allowed myself 1 small treat (300 calories or less)

today I exercised

○	○	○	○	○
15 mins.	30 mins.	45 mins.	60 mins.	More!

my workout was: _____

_____

my wins

_____

_____

_____

my struggles

_____

_____

_____

I took care of myself by

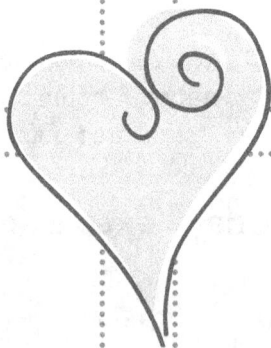

Week 3, Day 3

how I am feeling today . . .

today, I am grateful for

_____

_____

_____

_____

_____

my intention for tomorrow is:

. . . which helps me reach my weekly goal of:

. . . and helps me reach my master goal of:

my intention for tomorrow is:

. . . which helps me reach my weekly goal of:

. . . and helps me reach my master goal of:

my intention for tomorrow is:

. . . which helps me reach my weekly goal of:

. . . and helps me reach my master goal of:

today I ate

breakfast
- ○ 1-2 servings of fruit and/or veggies
- ○ 1 serving of whole grains
- ○ 1 serving of protein
- ○ drank water

snack
- ○ 1-2 servings of fruit and/or veggies
- ○ 1 serving of whole grains
- ○ 1 serving of protein
- ○ drank water

lunch
- ○ 1-2 servings of fruit and/or veggies
- ○ 1 serving of whole grains
- ○ 1 serving of protein
- ○ drank water

snack
- ○ 1-2 servings of fruit and/or veggies
- ○ 1 serving of whole grains
- ○ 1 serving of protein
- ○ drank water

dinner
- ○ 1-2 servings of fruit and/or veggies
- ○ 1 serving of whole grains
- ○ 1 serving of protein
- ○ drank water

snack
- ○ 1-2 servings of fruit and/or veggies
- ○ 1 serving of whole grains
- ○ 1 serving of protein
- ○ drank water

- ○ Ate every 2-3 hours
- ○ Stopped eating 3 hours before bed
- ○ Allowed myself 1 small treat (300 calories or less)

today I exercised

○ 15 mins.   ○ 30 mins.   ○ 45 mins.   ○ 60 mins.   ○ More!

my workout was: _____

_____

my wins

_____

_____

_____

my struggles

_____

_____

_____

I took care of myself by

how I am feeling today . . .

today, I am grateful for

_____

_____

_____

_____

_____

my intention for tomorrow is:

. . . which helps me reach my weekly goal of:

. . . and helps me reach my master goal of:

my intention for tomorrow is:

. . . which helps me reach my weekly goal of:

. . . and helps me reach my master goal of:

my intention for tomorrow is:

. . . which helps me reach my weekly goal of:

. . . and helps me reach my master goal of:

Week 3, Day 5

today I ate

breakfast
- ○ 1-2 servings of fruit and/or veggies
- ○ 1 serving of whole grains
- ○ 1 serving of protein
- ○ drank water

snack
- ○ 1-2 servings of fruit and/or veggies
- ○ 1 serving of whole grains
- ○ 1 serving of protein
- ○ drank water

lunch
- ○ 1-2 servings of fruit and/or veggies
- ○ 1 serving of whole grains
- ○ 1 serving of protein
- ○ drank water

snack
- ○ 1-2 servings of fruit and/or veggies
- ○ 1 serving of whole grains
- ○ 1 serving of protein
- ○ drank water

dinner
- ○ 1-2 servings of fruit and/or veggies
- ○ 1 serving of whole grains
- ○ 1 serving of protein
- ○ drank water

snack
- ○ 1-2 servings of fruit and/or veggies
- ○ 1 serving of whole grains
- ○ 1 serving of protein
- ○ drank water

- ○ Ate every 2-3 hours
- ○ Stopped eating 3 hours before bed
- ○ Allowed myself 1 small treat (300 calories or less)

today I exercised

○ 15 mins.   ○ 30 mins.   ○ 45 mins.   ○ 60 mins.   ○ More!

my workout was: _____

_____

my wins

_____

_____

_____

my struggles

_____

_____

_____

I took care of myself by

Week 3, Day 5

how I am feeling today . . .

today, I am grateful for

_____

_____

_____

_____

_____

my intention for tomorrow is:

. . . which helps me reach my weekly goal of:

. . . and helps me reach my master goal of:

my intention for tomorrow is:

. . . which helps me reach my weekly goal of:

. . . and helps me reach my master goal of:

my intention for tomorrow is:

. . . which helps me reach my weekly goal of:

. . . and helps me reach my master goal of:

Week 3, Day 6

today I ate

breakfast
- ○ 1-2 servings of fruit and/or veggies
- ○ 1 serving of whole grains
- ○ 1 serving of protein
- ○ drank water

snack
- ○ 1-2 servings of fruit and/or veggies
- ○ 1 serving of whole grains
- ○ 1 serving of protein
- ○ drank water

lunch
- ○ 1-2 servings of fruit and/or veggies
- ○ 1 serving of whole grains
- ○ 1 serving of protein
- ○ drank water

snack
- ○ 1-2 servings of fruit and/or veggies
- ○ 1 serving of whole grains
- ○ 1 serving of protein
- ○ drank water

dinner
- ○ 1-2 servings of fruit and/or veggies
- ○ 1 serving of whole grains
- ○ 1 serving of protein
- ○ drank water

snack
- ○ 1-2 servings of fruit and/or veggies
- ○ 1 serving of whole grains
- ○ 1 serving of protein
- ○ drank water

- ○ Ate every 2-3 hours
- ○ Stopped eating 3 hours before bed
- ○ Allowed myself 1 small treat (300 calories or less)

today I exercised

○ 15 mins.   ○ 30 mins.   ○ 45 mins.   ○ 60 mins.   ○ More!

my workout was: _____

_____

my wins	my struggles
_____	_____
_____	_____
_____	_____

I took care of myself by

Week 3, Day 6

how I am feeling today . . .

today, I am grateful for

_____

_____

_____

_____

_____

my intention for tomorrow is:

. . . which helps me reach my weekly goal of:

. . . and helps me reach my master goal of:

my intention for tomorrow is:

. . . which helps me reach my weekly goal of:

. . . and helps me reach my master goal of:

my intention for tomorrow is:

. . . which helps me reach my weekly goal of:

. . . and helps me reach my master goal of:

Week 3, Day 7

today I ate

breakfast
- ○ 1-2 servings of fruit and/or veggies
- ○ 1 serving of whole grains
- ○ 1 serving of protein
- ○ drank water

snack
- ○ 1-2 servings of fruit and/or veggies
- ○ 1 serving of whole grains
- ○ 1 serving of protein
- ○ drank water

lunch
- ○ 1-2 servings of fruit and/or veggies
- ○ 1 serving of whole grains
- ○ 1 serving of protein
- ○ drank water

snack
- ○ 1-2 servings of fruit and/or veggies
- ○ 1 serving of whole grains
- ○ 1 serving of protein
- ○ drank water

dinner
- ○ 1-2 servings of fruit and/or veggies
- ○ 1 serving of whole grains
- ○ 1 serving of protein
- ○ drank water

snack
- ○ 1-2 servings of fruit and/or veggies
- ○ 1 serving of whole grains
- ○ 1 serving of protein
- ○ drank water

○ Ate every 2-3 hours
○ Stopped eating 3 hours before bed
○ Allowed myself 1 small treat (300 calories or less)

today I exercised

○ 15 mins.   ○ 30 mins.   ○ 45 mins.   ○ 60 mins.   ○ More!

my workout was: _____

_____

my wins

_____

_____

_____

my struggles

_____

_____

_____

I took care of myself by

how I am feeling today . . .

today, I am grateful for

_____

_____

_____

_____

_____

my intention for tomorrow is:

. . . which helps me reach my weekly goal of:

. . . and helps me reach my master goal of:

my intention for tomorrow is:

. . . which helps me reach my weekly goal of:

. . . and helps me reach my master goal of:

my intention for tomorrow is:

. . . which helps me reach my weekly goal of:

. . . and helps me reach my master goal of:

Week 4, Day 1

today I ate

breakfast
- O 1-2 servings of fruit and/or veggies
- O 1 serving of whole grains
- O 1 serving of protein
- O drank water

snack
- O 1-2 servings of fruit and/or veggies
- O 1 serving of whole grains
- O 1 serving of protein
- O drank water

lunch
- O 1-2 servings of fruit and/or veggies
- O 1 serving of whole grains
- O 1 serving of protein
- O drank water

snack
- O 1-2 servings of fruit and/or veggies
- O 1 serving of whole grains
- O 1 serving of protein
- O drank water

dinner
- O 1-2 servings of fruit and/or veggies
- O 1 serving of whole grains
- O 1 serving of protein
- O drank water

snack
- O 1-2 servings of fruit and/or veggies
- O 1 serving of whole grains
- O 1 serving of protein
- O drank water

- O Ate every 2-3 hours
- O Stopped eating 3 hours before bed
- O Allowed myself 1 small treat (300 calories or less)

today I exercised

O	O	O	O	O
15 mins.	30 mins.	45 mins.	60 mins.	More!

my workout was: _____

_____

my wins

_____

_____

_____

my struggles

_____

_____

_____

I took care of myself by

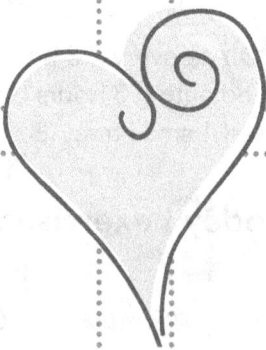

how I am feeling today . . .

today, I am grateful for

_____

_____

_____

_____

_____

my intention for tomorrow is:

. . . which helps me reach my weekly goal of:

. . . and helps me reach my master goal of:

my intention for tomorrow is:

. . . which helps me reach my weekly goal of:

. . . and helps me reach my master goal of:

my intention for tomorrow is:

. . . which helps me reach my weekly goal of:

. . . and helps me reach my master goal of:

Week 4, Day 2

today I ate

breakfast
- O 1-2 servings of fruit and/or veggies
- O 1 serving of whole grains
- O 1 serving of protein
- O drank water

snack
- O 1-2 servings of fruit and/or veggies
- O 1 serving of whole grains
- O 1 serving of protein
- O drank water

lunch
- O 1-2 servings of fruit and/or veggies
- O 1 serving of whole grains
- O 1 serving of protein
- O drank water

snack
- O 1-2 servings of fruit and/or veggies
- O 1 serving of whole grains
- O 1 serving of protein
- O drank water

dinner
- O 1-2 servings of fruit and/or veggies
- O 1 serving of whole grains
- O 1 serving of protein
- O drank water

snack
- O 1-2 servings of fruit and/or veggies
- O 1 serving of whole grains
- O 1 serving of protein
- O drank water

- O Ate every 2-3 hours
- O Stopped eating 3 hours before bed
- O Allowed myself 1 small treat (300 calories or less)

today I exercised

O 15 mins.   O 30 mins.   O 45 mins.   O 60 mins.   O More!

my workout was: _____

_____

my wins

_____

_____

_____

my struggles

_____

_____

_____

I took care of myself by

Week 4, Day 2

how I am feeling today . . .

today, I am grateful for

_____

_____

_____

_____

_____

my intention for tomorrow is:

. . . which helps me reach my weekly goal of:

. . . and helps me reach my master goal of:

my intention for tomorrow is:

. . . which helps me reach my weekly goal of:

. . . and helps me reach my master goal of:

my intention for tomorrow is:

. . . which helps me reach my weekly goal of:

. . . and helps me reach my master goal of:

Week 4, Day 3

today I ate

breakfast
- O 1-2 servings of fruit and/or veggies
- O 1 serving of whole grains
- O 1 serving of protein
- O drank water

snack
- O 1-2 servings of fruit and/or veggies
- O 1 serving of whole grains
- O 1 serving of protein
- O drank water

lunch
- O 1-2 servings of fruit and/or veggies
- O 1 serving of whole grains
- O 1 serving of protein
- O drank water

snack
- O 1-2 servings of fruit and/or veggies
- O 1 serving of whole grains
- O 1 serving of protein
- O drank water

dinner
- O 1-2 servings of fruit and/or veggies
- O 1 serving of whole grains
- O 1 serving of protein
- O drank water

snack
- O 1-2 servings of fruit and/or veggies
- O 1 serving of whole grains
- O 1 serving of protein
- O drank water

- O Ate every 2-3 hours
- O Stopped eating 3 hours before bed
- O Allowed myself 1 small treat (300 calories or less)

today I exercised

O 15 mins.   O 30 mins.   O 45 mins.   O 60 mins.   O More!

my workout was: _____

_____

my wins

_____

_____

_____

my struggles

_____

_____

_____

I took care of myself by

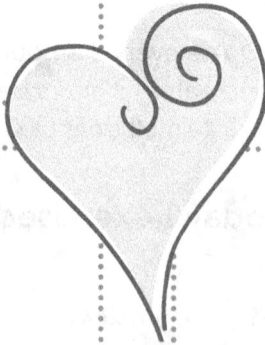

how I am feeling today . . .

today, I am grateful for

_____

_____

_____

_____

_____

my intention for tomorrow is:

. . . which helps me reach my weekly goal of:

. . . and helps me reach my master goal of:

my intention for tomorrow is:

. . . which helps me reach my weekly goal of:

. . . and helps me reach my master goal of:

my intention for tomorrow is:

. . . which helps me reach my weekly goal of:

. . . and helps me reach my master goal of:

Week 4, Day 4

today I ate

breakfast
- ○ 1-2 servings of fruit and/or veggies
- ○ 1 serving of whole grains
- ○ 1 serving of protein
- ○ drank water

snack
- ○ 1-2 servings of fruit and/or veggies
- ○ 1 serving of whole grains
- ○ 1 serving of protein
- ○ drank water

lunch
- ○ 1-2 servings of fruit and/or veggies
- ○ 1 serving of whole grains
- ○ 1 serving of protein
- ○ drank water

snack
- ○ 1-2 servings of fruit and/or veggies
- ○ 1 serving of whole grains
- ○ 1 serving of protein
- ○ drank water

dinner
- ○ 1-2 servings of fruit and/or veggies
- ○ 1 serving of whole grains
- ○ 1 serving of protein
- ○ drank water

snack
- ○ 1-2 servings of fruit and/or veggies
- ○ 1 serving of whole grains
- ○ 1 serving of protein
- ○ drank water

- ○ Ate every 2-3 hours
- ○ Stopped eating 3 hours before bed
- ○ Allowed myself 1 small treat (300 calories or less)

today I exercised

○	○	○	○	○
15 mins.	30 mins.	45 mins.	60 mins.	More!

my workout was: _____

_____

my wins

_____

_____

_____

my struggles

_____

_____

_____

I took care of myself by

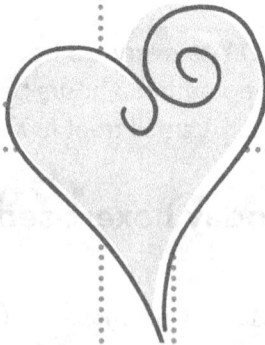

Week 4, Day 4

how I am feeling today . . .

today, I am grateful for

_____

_____

_____

_____

_____

my intention for tomorrow is:

. . . which helps me reach my weekly goal of:

. . . and helps me reach my master goal of:

my intention for tomorrow is:

. . . which helps me reach my weekly goal of:

. . . and helps me reach my master goal of:

my intention for tomorrow is:

. . . which helps me reach my weekly goal of:

. . . and helps me reach my master goal of:

Week 4, Day 5

today I ate

breakfast
- ○ 1-2 servings of fruit and/or veggies
- ○ 1 serving of whole grains
- ○ 1 serving of protein
- ○ drank water

snack
- ○ 1-2 servings of fruit and/or veggies
- ○ 1 serving of whole grains
- ○ 1 serving of protein
- ○ drank water

lunch
- ○ 1-2 servings of fruit and/or veggies
- ○ 1 serving of whole grains
- ○ 1 serving of protein
- ○ drank water

snack
- ○ 1-2 servings of fruit and/or veggies
- ○ 1 serving of whole grains
- ○ 1 serving of protein
- ○ drank water

dinner
- ○ 1-2 servings of fruit and/or veggies
- ○ 1 serving of whole grains
- ○ 1 serving of protein
- ○ drank water

snack
- ○ 1-2 servings of fruit and/or veggies
- ○ 1 serving of whole grains
- ○ 1 serving of protein
- ○ drank water

- ○ Ate every 2-3 hours
- ○ Stopped eating 3 hours before bed
- ○ Allowed myself 1 small treat (300 calories or less)

today I exercised

○ 15 mins.   ○ 30 mins.   ○ 45 mins.   ○ 60 mins.   ○ More!

my workout was: _____

_____

Week 4, Day 5

my wins

_____

_____

_____

my struggles

_____

_____

_____

I took care of myself by

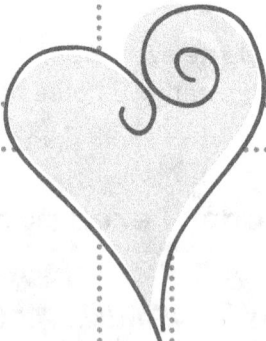

how I am feeling today . . .

today, I am grateful for

_____

_____

_____

_____

_____

my intention for tomorrow is:

. . . which helps me reach my weekly goal of:

. . . and helps me reach my master goal of:

my intention for tomorrow is:

. . . which helps me reach my weekly goal of:

. . . and helps me reach my master goal of:

my intention for tomorrow is:

. . . which helps me reach my weekly goal of:

. . . and helps me reach my master goal of:

today I ate

breakfast
- ○ 1-2 servings of fruit and/or veggies
- ○ 1 serving of whole grains
- ○ 1 serving of protein
- ○ drank water

snack
- ○ 1-2 servings of fruit and/or veggies
- ○ 1 serving of whole grains
- ○ 1 serving of protein
- ○ drank water

snack
- ○ 1-2 servings of fruit and/or veggies
- ○ 1 serving of whole grains
- ○ 1 serving of protein
- ○ drank water

dinner
- ○ 1-2 servings of fruit and/or veggies
- ○ 1 serving of whole grains
- ○ 1 serving of protein
- ○ drank water

lunch
- ○ 1-2 servings of fruit and/or veggies
- ○ 1 serving of whole grains
- ○ 1 serving of protein
- ○ drank water

snack
- ○ 1-2 servings of fruit and/or veggies
- ○ 1 serving of whole grains
- ○ 1 serving of protein
- ○ drank water

- ○ Ate every 2-3 hours
- ○ Stopped eating 3 hours before bed
- ○ Allowed myself 1 small treat (300 calories or less)

today I exercised

○ 15 mins.   ○ 30 mins.   ○ 45 mins.   ○ 60 mins.   ○ More!

my workout was: _____

_____

my wins

_____

_____

_____

my struggles

_____

_____

_____

I took care of myself by

how I am feeling today . . .

today, I am grateful for

_____

_____

_____

_____

_____

my intention for tomorrow is:

. . . which helps me reach my weekly goal of:

. . . and helps me reach my master goal of:

my intention for tomorrow is:

. . . which helps me reach my weekly goal of:

. . . and helps me reach my master goal of:

my intention for tomorrow is:

. . . which helps me reach my weekly goal of:

. . . and helps me reach my master goal of:

Week 4, Day 7

today I ate

breakfast
- ○ 1-2 servings of fruit and/or veggies
- ○ 1 serving of whole grains
- ○ 1 serving of protein
- ○ drank water

snack
- ○ 1-2 servings of fruit and/or veggies
- ○ 1 serving of whole grains
- ○ 1 serving of protein
- ○ drank water

lunch
- ○ 1-2 servings of fruit and/or veggies
- ○ 1 serving of whole grains
- ○ 1 serving of protein
- ○ drank water

snack
- ○ 1-2 servings of fruit and/or veggies
- ○ 1 serving of whole grains
- ○ 1 serving of protein
- ○ drank water

dinner
- ○ 1-2 servings of fruit and/or veggies
- ○ 1 serving of whole grains
- ○ 1 serving of protein
- ○ drank water

snack
- ○ 1-2 servings of fruit and/or veggies
- ○ 1 serving of whole grains
- ○ 1 serving of protein
- ○ drank water

- ○ Ate every 2-3 hours
- ○ Stopped eating 3 hours before bed
- ○ Allowed myself 1 small treat (300 calories or less)

today I exercised

○ 15 mins.   ○ 30 mins.   ○ 45 mins.   ○ 60 mins.   ○ More!

my workout was: _____

_____

Week 4, Day 7

my wins

_____

_____

_____

my struggles

_____

_____

_____

I took care of myself by

Week 4, Day 7

how I am feeling today . . .

today, I am grateful for

_____

_____

_____

_____

_____

my intention for tomorrow is:

. . . which helps me reach my weekly goal of:

. . . and helps me reach my master goal of:

my intention for tomorrow is:

. . . which helps me reach my weekly goal of:

. . . and helps me reach my master goal of:

my intention for tomorrow is:

. . . which helps me reach my weekly goal of:

. . . and helps me reach my master goal of:

Week 5, Day 1

today I ate

breakfast
- ○ 1-2 servings of fruit and/or veggies
- ○ 1 serving of whole grains
- ○ 1 serving of protein
- ○ drank water

snack
- ○ 1-2 servings of fruit and/or veggies
- ○ 1 serving of whole grains
- ○ 1 serving of protein
- ○ drank water

lunch
- ○ 1-2 servings of fruit and/or veggies
- ○ 1 serving of whole grains
- ○ 1 serving of protein
- ○ drank water

snack
- ○ 1-2 servings of fruit and/or veggies
- ○ 1 serving of whole grains
- ○ 1 serving of protein
- ○ drank water

dinner
- ○ 1-2 servings of fruit and/or veggies
- ○ 1 serving of whole grains
- ○ 1 serving of protein
- ○ drank water

snack
- ○ 1-2 servings of fruit and/or veggies
- ○ 1 serving of whole grains
- ○ 1 serving of protein
- ○ drank water

- ○ Ate every 2-3 hours
- ○ Stopped eating 3 hours before bed
- ○ Allowed myself 1 small treat (300 calories or less)

today I exercised

○ 15 mins. ○ 30 mins. ○ 45 mins. ○ 60 mins. ○ More!

my workout was: _____

_____

Week 5, Day 1

my wins

_____

_____

_____

my struggles

_____

_____

_____

I took care of myself by

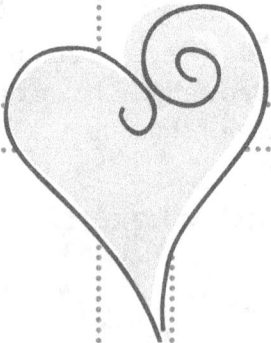

how I am feeling today . . .

today, I am grateful for

_____

_____

_____

_____

_____

my intention for tomorrow is:

. . . which helps me reach my weekly goal of:

. . . and helps me reach my master goal of:

my intention for tomorrow is:

. . . which helps me reach my weekly goal of:

. . . and helps me reach my master goal of:

my intention for tomorrow is:

. . . which helps me reach my weekly goal of:

. . . and helps me reach my master goal of:

Week 5, Day 2

today I ate

breakfast
- ○ 1-2 servings of fruit and/or veggies
- ○ 1 serving of whole grains
- ○ 1 serving of protein
- ○ drank water

snack
- ○ 1-2 servings of fruit and/or veggies
- ○ 1 serving of whole grains
- ○ 1 serving of protein
- ○ drank water

lunch
- ○ 1-2 servings of fruit and/or veggies
- ○ 1 serving of whole grains
- ○ 1 serving of protein
- ○ drank water

snack
- ○ 1-2 servings of fruit and/or veggies
- ○ 1 serving of whole grains
- ○ 1 serving of protein
- ○ drank water

dinner
- ○ 1-2 servings of fruit and/or veggies
- ○ 1 serving of whole grains
- ○ 1 serving of protein
- ○ drank water

snack
- ○ 1-2 servings of fruit and/or veggies
- ○ 1 serving of whole grains
- ○ 1 serving of protein
- ○ drank water

- ○ Ate every 2-3 hours
- ○ Stopped eating 3 hours before bed
- ○ Allowed myself 1 small treat (300 calories or less)

today I exercised

○ 15 mins. ○ 30 mins. ○ 45 mins. ○ 60 mins. ○ More!

my workout was: _____

_____

my wins

_____

_____

_____

❀

my struggles

_____

_____

_____

❀

I took care of myself by

Week 5, Day 2

how I am feeling today . . .

today, I am grateful for

_____

_____

_____

_____

_____

my intention for tomorrow is:

. . . which helps me reach my weekly goal of:

. . . and helps me reach my master goal of:

my intention for tomorrow is:

. . . which helps me reach my weekly goal of:

. . . and helps me reach my master goal of:

my intention for tomorrow is:

. . . which helps me reach my weekly goal of:

. . . and helps me reach my master goal of:

today I ate

breakfast
- ○ 1-2 servings of fruit and/or veggies
- ○ 1 serving of whole grains
- ○ 1 serving of protein
- ○ drank water

snack
- ○ 1-2 servings of fruit and/or veggies
- ○ 1 serving of whole grains
- ○ 1 serving of protein
- ○ drank water

snack
- ○ 1-2 servings of fruit and/or veggies
- ○ 1 serving of whole grains
- ○ 1 serving of protein
- ○ drank water

dinner
- ○ 1-2 servings of fruit and/or veggies
- ○ 1 serving of whole grains
- ○ 1 serving of protein
- ○ drank water

lunch
- ○ 1-2 servings of fruit and/or veggies
- ○ 1 serving of whole grains
- ○ 1 serving of protein
- ○ drank water

snack
- ○ 1-2 servings of fruit and/or veggies
- ○ 1 serving of whole grains
- ○ 1 serving of protein
- ○ drank water

- ○ Ate every 2-3 hours
- ○ Stopped eating 3 hours before bed
- ○ Allowed myself 1 small treat (300 calories or less)

today I exercised

○	○	○	○	○
15 mins.	30 mins.	45 mins.	60 mins.	More!

my workout was: _____

_____

Week 5, Day 3

my wins

my struggles

I took care of myself by

how I am feeling today . . .

today, I am grateful for

_____

_____

_____

_____

_____

my intention for tomorrow is:

. . . which helps me reach my weekly goal of:

. . . and helps me reach my master goal of:

my intention for tomorrow is:

. . . which helps me reach my weekly goal of:

. . . and helps me reach my master goal of:

my intention for tomorrow is:

. . . which helps me reach my weekly goal of:

. . . and helps me reach my master goal of:

Week 5, Day 4

today I ate

breakfast
- ○ 1-2 servings of fruit and/or veggies
- ○ 1 serving of whole grains
- ○ 1 serving of protein
- ○ drank water

snack
- ○ 1-2 servings of fruit and/or veggies
- ○ 1 serving of whole grains
- ○ 1 serving of protein
- ○ drank water

lunch
- ○ 1-2 servings of fruit and/or veggies
- ○ 1 serving of whole grains
- ○ 1 serving of protein
- ○ drank water

snack
- ○ 1-2 servings of fruit and/or veggies
- ○ 1 serving of whole grains
- ○ 1 serving of protein
- ○ drank water

dinner
- ○ 1-2 servings of fruit and/or veggies
- ○ 1 serving of whole grains
- ○ 1 serving of protein
- ○ drank water

snack
- ○ 1-2 servings of fruit and/or veggies
- ○ 1 serving of whole grains
- ○ 1 serving of protein
- ○ drank water

- ○ Ate every 2-3 hours
- ○ Stopped eating 3 hours before bed
- ○ Allowed myself 1 small treat (300 calories or less)

today I exercised

○ 15 mins.   ○ 30 mins.   ○ 45 mins.   ○ 60 mins.   ○ More!

my workout was: _____

_____

Week 5, Day 4

my wins	my struggles
_____	_____
_____	_____
_____	_____

I took care of myself by

how I am feeling today . . .

today, I am grateful for

_____

_____

_____

_____

_____

my intention for tomorrow is:

. . . which helps me reach my weekly goal of:

. . . and helps me reach my master goal of:

my intention for tomorrow is:

. . . which helps me reach my weekly goal of:

. . . and helps me reach my master goal of:

my intention for tomorrow is:

. . . which helps me reach my weekly goal of:

. . . and helps me reach my master goal of:

today I ate

breakfast
- ○ 1-2 servings of fruit and/or veggies
- ○ 1 serving of whole grains
- ○ 1 serving of protein
- ○ drank water

snack
- ○ 1-2 servings of fruit and/or veggies
- ○ 1 serving of whole grains
- ○ 1 serving of protein
- ○ drank water

snack
- ○ 1-2 servings of fruit and/or veggies
- ○ 1 serving of whole grains
- ○ 1 serving of protein
- ○ drank water

dinner
- ○ 1-2 servings of fruit and/or veggies
- ○ 1 serving of whole grains
- ○ 1 serving of protein
- ○ drank water

lunch
- ○ 1-2 servings of fruit and/or veggies
- ○ 1 serving of whole grains
- ○ 1 serving of protein
- ○ drank water

snack
- ○ 1-2 servings of fruit and/or veggies
- ○ 1 serving of whole grains
- ○ 1 serving of protein
- ○ drank water

- ○ Ate every 2-3 hours
- ○ Stopped eating 3 hours before bed
- ○ Allowed myself 1 small treat (300 calories or less)

today I exercised

○	○	○	○	○
15 mins.	30 mins.	45 mins.	60 mins.	More!

my workout was: _____
_____

Week 5, Day 5

my wins

_____

_____

_____

my struggles

_____

_____

_____

I took care of myself by

Week 5, Day 5

how I am feeling today . . .

today, I am grateful for

_____

_____

_____

_____

_____

my intention for tomorrow is:

. . . which helps me reach my weekly goal of:

. . . and helps me reach my master goal of:

my intention for tomorrow is:

. . . which helps me reach my weekly goal of:

. . . and helps me reach my master goal of:

my intention for tomorrow is:

. . . which helps me reach my weekly goal of:

. . . and helps me reach my master goal of:

Week 5, Day 6

today I ate

breakfast
- ○ 1-2 servings of fruit and/or veggies
- ○ 1 serving of whole grains
- ○ 1 serving of protein
- ○ drank water

snack
- ○ 1-2 servings of fruit and/or veggies
- ○ 1 serving of whole grains
- ○ 1 serving of protein
- ○ drank water

lunch
- ○ 1-2 servings of fruit and/or veggies
- ○ 1 serving of whole grains
- ○ 1 serving of protein
- ○ drank water

snack
- ○ 1-2 servings of fruit and/or veggies
- ○ 1 serving of whole grains
- ○ 1 serving of protein
- ○ drank water

dinner
- ○ 1-2 servings of fruit and/or veggies
- ○ 1 serving of whole grains
- ○ 1 serving of protein
- ○ drank water

snack
- ○ 1-2 servings of fruit and/or veggies
- ○ 1 serving of whole grains
- ○ 1 serving of protein
- ○ drank water

- ○ Ate every 2-3 hours
- ○ Stopped eating 3 hours before bed
- ○ Allowed myself 1 small treat (300 calories or less)

today I exercised

○ 15 mins.   ○ 30 mins.   ○ 45 mins.   ○ 60 mins.   ○ More!

my workout was: _____

_____

my wins

_____

_____

_____

my struggles

_____

_____

_____

I took care of myself by

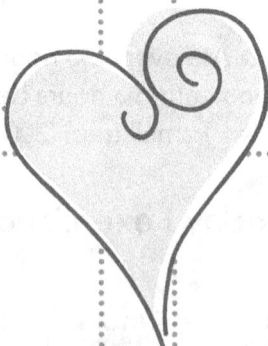

how I am feeling today . . .

today, I am grateful for

_____

_____

_____

_____

_____

my intention for tomorrow is:

. . . which helps me reach my weekly goal of:

. . . and helps me reach my master goal of:

my intention for tomorrow is:

. . . which helps me reach my weekly goal of:

. . . and helps me reach my master goal of:

my intention for tomorrow is:

. . . which helps me reach my weekly goal of:

. . . and helps me reach my master goal of:

Week 5, Day 7

today I ate

breakfast
- ○ 1-2 servings of fruit and/or veggies
- ○ 1 serving of whole grains
- ○ 1 serving of protein
- ○ drank water

snack
- ○ 1-2 servings of fruit and/or veggies
- ○ 1 serving of whole grains
- ○ 1 serving of protein
- ○ drank water

lunch
- ○ 1-2 servings of fruit and/or veggies
- ○ 1 serving of whole grains
- ○ 1 serving of protein
- ○ drank water

snack
- ○ 1-2 servings of fruit and/or veggies
- ○ 1 serving of whole grains
- ○ 1 serving of protein
- ○ drank water

dinner
- ○ 1-2 servings of fruit and/or veggies
- ○ 1 serving of whole grains
- ○ 1 serving of protein
- ○ drank water

snack
- ○ 1-2 servings of fruit and/or veggies
- ○ 1 serving of whole grains
- ○ 1 serving of protein
- ○ drank water

- ○ Ate every 2-3 hours
- ○ Stopped eating 3 hours before bed
- ○ Allowed myself 1 small treat (300 calories or less)

today I exercised

○ 15 mins.   ○ 30 mins.   ○ 45 mins.   ○ 60 mins.   ○ More!

my workout was: _____
_____

Week 5, Day 7

my wins

_____

_____

_____

my struggles

_____

_____

_____

I took care of myself by

how I am feeling today . . .

today, I am grateful for

_____

_____

_____

_____

_____

my intention for tomorrow is:

. . . which helps me reach my weekly goal of:

. . . and helps me reach my master goal of:

my intention for tomorrow is:

. . . which helps me reach my weekly goal of:

. . . and helps me reach my master goal of:

my intention for tomorrow is:

. . . which helps me reach my weekly goal of:

. . . and helps me reach my master goal of:

Week 6, Day 1

today I ate

breakfast
- ○ 1-2 servings of fruit and/or veggies
- ○ 1 serving of whole grains
- ○ 1 serving of protein
- ○ drank water

snack
- ○ 1-2 servings of fruit and/or veggies
- ○ 1 serving of whole grains
- ○ 1 serving of protein
- ○ drank water

lunch
- ○ 1-2 servings of fruit and/or veggies
- ○ 1 serving of whole grains
- ○ 1 serving of protein
- ○ drank water

snack
- ○ 1-2 servings of fruit and/or veggies
- ○ 1 serving of whole grains
- ○ 1 serving of protein
- ○ drank water

dinner
- ○ 1-2 servings of fruit and/or veggies
- ○ 1 serving of whole grains
- ○ 1 serving of protein
- ○ drank water

snack
- ○ 1-2 servings of fruit and/or veggies
- ○ 1 serving of whole grains
- ○ 1 serving of protein
- ○ drank water

- ○ Ate every 2-3 hours
- ○ Stopped eating 3 hours before bed
- ○ Allowed myself 1 small treat (300 calories or less)

today I exercised

○ 15 mins.   ○ 30 mins.   ○ 45 mins.   ○ 60 mins.   ○ More!

my workout was: _____

_____

my wins

_____

_____

_____

my struggles

_____

_____

_____

I took care of myself by

how I am feeling today . . .

today, I am grateful for

_____

_____

_____

_____

_____

my intention for tomorrow is:

. . . which helps me reach my weekly goal of:

. . . and helps me reach my master goal of:

my intention for tomorrow is:

. . . which helps me reach my weekly goal of:

. . . and helps me reach my master goal of:

my intention for tomorrow is:

. . . which helps me reach my weekly goal of:

. . . and helps me reach my master goal of:

Week 6, Day 2

today I ate

breakfast
- ○ 1-2 servings of fruit and/or veggies
- ○ 1 serving of whole grains
- ○ 1 serving of protein
- ○ drank water

snack
- ○ 1-2 servings of fruit and/or veggies
- ○ 1 serving of whole grains
- ○ 1 serving of protein
- ○ drank water

snack
- ○ 1-2 servings of fruit and/or veggies
- ○ 1 serving of whole grains
- ○ 1 serving of protein
- ○ drank water

dinner
- ○ 1-2 servings of fruit and/or veggies
- ○ 1 serving of whole grains
- ○ 1 serving of protein
- ○ drank water

lunch
- ○ 1-2 servings of fruit and/or veggies
- ○ 1 serving of whole grains
- ○ 1 serving of protein
- ○ drank water

snack
- ○ 1-2 servings of fruit and/or veggies
- ○ 1 serving of whole grains
- ○ 1 serving of protein
- ○ drank water

- ○ Ate every 2-3 hours
- ○ Stopped eating 3 hours before bed
- ○ Allowed myself 1 small treat (300 calories or less)

today I exercised

○	○	○	○	○
15 mins.	30 mins.	45 mins.	60 mins.	More!

my workout was: _____

_____

Week 6, Day 2

my wins

_____

_____

_____

❃

my struggles

_____

_____

_____

❃

I took care of myself by

Week 6, Day 2

how I am feeling today . . .

today, I am grateful for

_____

_____

_____

_____

_____

my intention for tomorrow is:

. . . which helps me reach my weekly goal of:

. . . and helps me reach my master goal of:

my intention for tomorrow is:

. . . which helps me reach my weekly goal of:

. . . and helps me reach my master goal of:

my intention for tomorrow is:

. . . which helps me reach my weekly goal of:

. . . and helps me reach my master goal of:

Week 6, Day 3

today I ate

breakfast
- ○ 1-2 servings of fruit and/or veggies
- ○ 1 serving of whole grains
- ○ 1 serving of protein
- ○ drank water

snack
- ○ 1-2 servings of fruit and/or veggies
- ○ 1 serving of whole grains
- ○ 1 serving of protein
- ○ drank water

lunch
- ○ 1-2 servings of fruit and/or veggies
- ○ 1 serving of whole grains
- ○ 1 serving of protein
- ○ drank water

snack
- ○ 1-2 servings of fruit and/or veggies
- ○ 1 serving of whole grains
- ○ 1 serving of protein
- ○ drank water

dinner
- ○ 1-2 servings of fruit and/or veggies
- ○ 1 serving of whole grains
- ○ 1 serving of protein
- ○ drank water

snack
- ○ 1-2 servings of fruit and/or veggies
- ○ 1 serving of whole grains
- ○ 1 serving of protein
- ○ drank water

- ○ Ate every 2-3 hours
- ○ Stopped eating 3 hours before bed
- ○ Allowed myself 1 small treat (300 calories or less)

today I exercised

○ 15 mins.   ○ 30 mins.   ○ 45 mins.   ○ 60 mins.   ○ More!

my workout was: _____

_____

my wins	my struggles
_____	_____
_____	_____
_____	_____

I took care of myself by

how I am feeling today . . .

today, I am grateful for

_____

_____

_____

_____

_____

my intention for tomorrow is:

. . . which helps me reach my weekly goal of:

. . . and helps me reach my master goal of:

my intention for tomorrow is:

. . . which helps me reach my weekly goal of:

. . . and helps me reach my master goal of:

my intention for tomorrow is:

. . . which helps me reach my weekly goal of:

. . . and helps me reach my master goal of:

Week 6, Day 4

today I ate

breakfast
- ○ 1-2 servings of fruit and/or veggies
- ○ 1 serving of whole grains
- ○ 1 serving of protein
- ○ drank water

snack
- ○ 1-2 servings of fruit and/or veggies
- ○ 1 serving of whole grains
- ○ 1 serving of protein
- ○ drank water

lunch
- ○ 1-2 servings of fruit and/or veggies
- ○ 1 serving of whole grains
- ○ 1 serving of protein
- ○ drank water

snack
- ○ 1-2 servings of fruit and/or veggies
- ○ 1 serving of whole grains
- ○ 1 serving of protein
- ○ drank water

dinner
- ○ 1-2 servings of fruit and/or veggies
- ○ 1 serving of whole grains
- ○ 1 serving of protein
- ○ drank water

snack
- ○ 1-2 servings of fruit and/or veggies
- ○ 1 serving of whole grains
- ○ 1 serving of protein
- ○ drank water

- ○ Ate every 2-3 hours
- ○ Stopped eating 3 hours before bed
- ○ Allowed myself 1 small treat (300 calories or less)

today I exercised

○	○	○	○	○
15 mins.	30 mins.	45 mins.	60 mins.	More!

my workout was: _____

_____

Week 6, Day 4

my wins

_____

_____

_____

my struggles

_____

_____

_____

I took care of myself by

Week 6, Day 4

how I am feeling today . . .

today, I am grateful for

_____

_____

_____

_____

_____

my intention for tomorrow is:

. . . which helps me reach my weekly goal of:

. . . and helps me reach my master goal of:

my intention for tomorrow is:

. . . which helps me reach my weekly goal of:

. . . and helps me reach my master goal of:

my intention for tomorrow is:

. . . which helps me reach my weekly goal of:

. . . and helps me reach my master goal of:

Week 6, Day 5

today I ate

breakfast
- ○ 1-2 servings of fruit and/or veggies
- ○ 1 serving of whole grains
- ○ 1 serving of protein
- ○ drank water

snack
- ○ 1-2 servings of fruit and/or veggies
- ○ 1 serving of whole grains
- ○ 1 serving of protein
- ○ drank water

lunch
- ○ 1-2 servings of fruit and/or veggies
- ○ 1 serving of whole grains
- ○ 1 serving of protein
- ○ drank water

snack
- ○ 1-2 servings of fruit and/or veggies
- ○ 1 serving of whole grains
- ○ 1 serving of protein
- ○ drank water

dinner
- ○ 1-2 servings of fruit and/or veggies
- ○ 1 serving of whole grains
- ○ 1 serving of protein
- ○ drank water

snack
- ○ 1-2 servings of fruit and/or veggies
- ○ 1 serving of whole grains
- ○ 1 serving of protein
- ○ drank water

- ○ Ate every 2-3 hours
- ○ Stopped eating 3 hours before bed
- ○ Allowed myself 1 small treat (300 calories or less)

today I exercised

○ 15 mins.   ○ 30 mins.   ○ 45 mins.   ○ 60 mins.   ○ More!

my workout was: _____

_____

my wins

_____

_____

_____

my struggles

_____

_____

_____

I took care of myself by

Week 6, Day 5

how I am feeling today . . .

today, I am grateful for

_____

_____

_____

_____

_____

my intention for tomorrow is:

. . . which helps me reach my weekly goal of:

. . . and helps me reach my master goal of:

my intention for tomorrow is:

. . . which helps me reach my weekly goal of:

. . . and helps me reach my master goal of:

my intention for tomorrow is:

. . . which helps me reach my weekly goal of:

. . . and helps me reach my master goal of:

Week 6, Day 6

today I ate

breakfast
- ○ 1-2 servings of fruit and/or veggies
- ○ 1 serving of whole grains
- ○ 1 serving of protein
- ○ drank water

snack
- ○ 1-2 servings of fruit and/or veggies
- ○ 1 serving of whole grains
- ○ 1 serving of protein
- ○ drank water

lunch
- ○ 1-2 servings of fruit and/or veggies
- ○ 1 serving of whole grains
- ○ 1 serving of protein
- ○ drank water

snack
- ○ 1-2 servings of fruit and/or veggies
- ○ 1 serving of whole grains
- ○ 1 serving of protein
- ○ drank water

dinner
- ○ 1-2 servings of fruit and/or veggies
- ○ 1 serving of whole grains
- ○ 1 serving of protein
- ○ drank water

snack
- ○ 1-2 servings of fruit and/or veggies
- ○ 1 serving of whole grains
- ○ 1 serving of protein
- ○ drank water

- ○ Ate every 2-3 hours
- ○ Stopped eating 3 hours before bed
- ○ Allowed myself 1 small treat (300 calories or less)

today I exercised

○ 15 mins.   ○ 30 mins.   ○ 45 mins.   ○ 60 mins.   ○ More!

my workout was: _____

_____

my wins

_____

_____

_____

my struggles

_____

_____

_____

I took care of myself by

how I am feeling today . . .

today, I am grateful for

_____

_____

_____

_____

_____

my intention for tomorrow is:

. . . which helps me reach my weekly goal of:

. . . and helps me reach my master goal of:

my intention for tomorrow is:

. . . which helps me reach my weekly goal of:

. . . and helps me reach my master goal of:

my intention for tomorrow is:

. . . which helps me reach my weekly goal of:

. . . and helps me reach my master goal of:

Week 6, Day 7

today I ate

breakfast
- ○ 1-2 servings of fruit and/or veggies
- ○ 1 serving of whole grains
- ○ 1 serving of protein
- ○ drank water

snack
- ○ 1-2 servings of fruit and/or veggies
- ○ 1 serving of whole grains
- ○ 1 serving of protein
- ○ drank water

snack
- ○ 1-2 servings of fruit and/or veggies
- ○ 1 serving of whole grains
- ○ 1 serving of protein
- ○ drank water

dinner
- ○ 1-2 servings of fruit and/or veggies
- ○ 1 serving of whole grains
- ○ 1 serving of protein
- ○ drank water

lunch
- ○ 1-2 servings of fruit and/or veggies
- ○ 1 serving of whole grains
- ○ 1 serving of protein
- ○ drank water

snack
- ○ 1-2 servings of fruit and/or veggies
- ○ 1 serving of whole grains
- ○ 1 serving of protein
- ○ drank water

- ○ Ate every 2-3 hours
- ○ Stopped eating 3 hours before bed
- ○ Allowed myself 1 small treat (300 calories or less)

today I exercised

○ 15 mins.   ○ 30 mins.   ○ 45 mins.   ○ 60 mins.   ○ More!

my workout was: _____

_____

Week 6, Day 7

my wins

_____

_____

_____

❀

my struggles

_____

_____

_____

❀

I took care of myself by

how I am feeling today . . .

today, I am grateful for

_____

_____

_____

_____

_____

my intention for tomorrow is:

. . . which helps me reach my weekly goal of:

. . . and helps me reach my master goal of:

my intention for tomorrow is:

. . . which helps me reach my weekly goal of:

. . . and helps me reach my master goal of:

my intention for tomorrow is:

. . . which helps me reach my weekly goal of:

. . . and helps me reach my master goal of:

How Far I've Come!

my current weight _____

my current measurements:

Left arm: _____

Right arm: _____

Chest: _____

Waist: _____

Hips: _____

Left thigh: _____

Right thigh: _____

I lost _____ pounds in six weeks!

I lost _____ inches in six weeks!

looking back, my greatest accomplishment during the past six weeks was:

Congratulations!
You Did a Great Job!

I hope you have found the past six weeks to
be the most rewarding of your life! By now,
you are feeling, and looking better than ever.

Now, it's time to get another copy of
this journal and continue on with your journey—
this time changing your body even more.

While you're at the bookstore, be sure to
take a look at the other titles available from
Scorpio Moon Publishing. We have several,
all of which will help you live a better life.

If you would like to receive daily motivation,
support from others who are using the
"In Just 6 Weeks" journal, and receive free journal
updates, please visit: InJust6Weeks.com.

www.ingramcontent.com/pod-product-compliance
Lightning Source LLC
Chambersburg PA
CBHW060851280326
41934CB00007B/1005